FUEL YOUR MUSCLES

The Essential Bodybuilding Diet for Women

MITT Creations

Table of Contents

Chapter 10:

Introduction

For women looking to build muscle and achieve their bodybuilding goals, having a proper diet is essential. A bodybuilding diet for women should be tailored to meet their individual needs and goals, taking into account their body type, activity level, and overall health. Eating the right foods in the right amounts can help fuel workouts, promote muscle growth, and ensure long-term health and wellness. With so many diet options out there, it can be difficult to figure out what works best. Here, we'll provide an overview of the best bodybuilding diet for women, along with tips and advice to get you started.

Chapter 1

Overview of Bodybuilding Nutrition for Women

Bodybuilding nutrition for women requires a specific approach to ensure the best results. It involves eating the right types of foods in the right amounts and timing meals to optimize the body's metabolism. Eating a balanced diet is key to providing the nutrients and energy needed to build muscle and lose fat. A diet that has adequate amounts of protein, healthy fats, complex carbohydrates, vitamins and minerals is essential to provide the energy, nutrients and micronutrients needed to support muscle growth and fat loss. For women bodybuilding nutrition, it is important to eat regularly throughout the day. Eating several small meals per day helps keep energy levels consistent and keeps the body's metabolism running optimally. Protein is essential for muscle growth and should be the main focus of a bodybuilding nutrition plan for women. Eating a variety of protein sources such as lean meats, fish, eggs, dairy, legumes and nuts provides the body with the necessary building blocks for muscle growth. In addition to protein, healthy fats are also important for bodybuilding nutrition. Healthy fats provide the body with essential fatty acids and help to fuel the body and support muscle growth. Eating nuts, avocados, olive oil and fatty fish are great sources of healthy fats. Complex carbohydrates should also be part of a bodybuilding nutrition plan for women. Foods such as oats, quinoa, sweet potatoes, brown rice and whole grains provide the body with slow-release energy and essential vitamins and minerals. Finally, it's important to make sure bodybuilding nutrition for women includes plenty of fresh fruits and vegetables to provide the body with essential vitamins, minerals and antioxidants. Eating a variety of fresh, whole foods is the best way to ensure the body is getting all the nutrients it needs. Bodybuilding nutrition for women can be a challenge, but with the right approach and the right foods, women can achieve the results they desire. Eating a balanced diet and timing meals to optimize the body's metabolism are essential for success.

Chapter 2

Protein and Macronutrients

Protein and macronutrients are incredibly important for any bodybuilding diet, especially for women. Protein is an essential component of muscle growth and repair, as well as providing fuel for the body during exercise. Macronutrients, such as carbohydrates, fats, and proteins, provide the primary sources of energy for the body. Getting the correct amount of these macronutrients is essential for women who are bodybuilding to maximize their results and stay healthy. Protein is the most important macronutrient for bodybuilders. It helps build muscle, repair tissue, and provides energy. It's also important for preserving lean body mass during a cutting phase. Women should aim to get at least 1.2 to 2.0 grams of protein per kilogram of bodyweight per day. Good sources of protein include lean meats, poultry, fish, eggs, dairy, nuts, and beans. Carbohydrates are the body's preferred source of energy and are necessary for fueling workouts. Eating an adequate amount of carbohydrates helps to replenish glycogen stores and support muscle growth. Women should aim for 3 to 4.5 grams of carbohydrates per kilogram of bodyweight per day. Good sources of carbohydrates include whole grains, fruits, vegetables, and legumes. Fats are an essential part of any diet and are necessary for hormone production, energy, and absorption of fat-soluble vitamins. Women should aim for .6 to 1.2 grams of fat per kilogram of bodyweight per day. Good sources of fat include nuts, seeds, avocados, extra-virgin olive oil, and fatty fish. By getting adequate amounts of protein and macronutrients, women can reach their bodybuilding goals and stay healthy. Eating a balanced diet full of nutritious foods is the best approach for any bodybuilder. Additionally, drinking enough water and staying hydrated is another important factor in maintaining health and achieving success.

Chapter 3

Carbohydrates

Carbohydrates are an important and essential part of a bodybuilding diet for women. Carbohydrates are the main source of energy for the body and are required to fuel muscle growth and development. They provide energy for the muscles to perform at their best and can also help with weight loss. Carbohydrates can be found in a variety of foods, including fruits, vegetables, grains, and dairy products. When it comes to bodybuilding, the type of carbohydrates you choose to eat will depend on your goals. Women bodybuilders should focus on complex carbohydrates that are low in fat and high in fiber. This will help to ensure that you are getting the necessary energy to power your workouts and the necessary nutrients to build muscle. Complex carbohydrates such as whole grains, legumes, quinoa, and oats will provide you with long-lasting energy and help to keep your blood sugar levels stable throughout the day. Whole grains are also high in fiber and B vitamins, which are important for muscle growth. Legumes are a great source of plant-based protein, as well as fiber and minerals. Quinoa is high in both protein and fiber and is an excellent choice for bodybuilding. Fruits and vegetables are also an important part of a bodybuilding diet for women. Fruits and vegetables provide essential vitamins, minerals, and antioxidants that can help with muscle recovery and growth. Fruits and vegetables are also low in calories and are a great source of fiber. Berries, oranges, apples, and dark leafy greens are all excellent choices for bodybuilding. Dairy products are also an important part of a bodybuilding diet for women. Dairy products contain protein and calcium, both of which are essential for muscle growth and development. Dairy products are also a great source of vitamin D, which helps to improve bone health. Low-fat dairy products such as Greek yogurt and skim milk are the best choices for bodybuilding. By including the right carbohydrates in your bodybuilding diet, you can ensure that you are getting the energy and nutrients you need to power your workouts and build muscle. Complex carbohydrates, fruits, vegetables, and dairy products are all important components of a bodybuilding diet for women. Be sure to incorporate these foods into your meals and snacks to ensure that you are getting the necessary energy and nutrients to fuel your workouts and reach your bodybuilding goals.

Chapter 4

Fats

When it comes to body building for women, fat is often overlooked, yet it plays an important role in a healthy diet. Fats provide essential fatty acids, which help to build up and maintain cell membranes, as well as provide a source of energy. In addition, fat helps to keep you full and can help you to reach your body building goals. Fat should be consumed in moderation and there are certain types of fat that are healthier than others. Unsaturated fat, such as olive oil, is a great choice. It can help to reduce inflammation and lower cholesterol levels. Monounsaturated fats, like those found in nuts and avocados, are also beneficial. Trans fats should be completely avoided as they can increase bad cholesterol levels and cause inflammation. It's also important to limit your intake of saturated fats, such as those found in red meat and dairy products. It's important to remember that fat should not be completely eliminated from your diet. Including healthy fats in your body building diet can help you to reach your goals. Healthy fats can also provide essential nutrients and can help to regulate hormones. In addition to providing essential fatty acids, healthy fats can also help to improve your overall health. They can help to reduce your risk of heart disease, stroke and diabetes, as well as improve your skin health. Some studies have also found that healthy fats can help to reduce the risk of certain types of cancer. To ensure that you are getting enough healthy fats in your diet, it's important to include them in your meals. Healthy fats can be added to salads and smoothies, or used to cook with. You can also use them as a topping for oatmeal or yogurt. Including healthy fats in your body building diet for women is essential for overall health and to help you reach your goals. Eating healthy fats can help to boost your energy levels and keep you feeling full for longer. So, don't be afraid to include healthy fats in your diet.

Chapter 5

Vitamins and Minerals

When it comes to bodybuilding, diet is key. Eating the right foods and maintaining a balanced diet is essential for anyone looking to sculpt their body and build muscle. Women bodybuilders, in particular, need to make sure they are getting all the essential vitamins and minerals their bodies need to build muscle, stay healthy, and perform at their peak. Vitamins are essential for healthy body function and optimal performance. Vitamin A, for example, helps keep the immune system strong and helps promote healthy vision. Vitamin B complex helps maintain healthy skin and eyes, while Vitamin C can help fight off infection and is necessary for energy production. Vitamin D is important for healthy bones and immune system, while vitamin E helps protect cells from damage and boosts metabolism. Minerals are also important for bodybuilding, as they are necessary for muscle growth and development. Calcium helps with muscle contraction and is important for healthy bones and teeth. Iron helps the body absorb and use oxygen and is essential for energy production. Magnesium helps with muscle contraction and helps the body use energy more efficiently, while zinc helps with wound healing and helps the body absorb vitamins and minerals. It is important for women bodybuilders to get enough of these essential vitamins and minerals in their diet. Eating a variety of fruits, vegetables, and lean proteins is the best way to ensure that your body is getting all the nutrients it needs to build muscle and stay healthy. Eating enough healthy fats such as olive oil and avocados can also help provide the body with essential fatty acids. Taking a multivitamin can also be beneficial, as it can help make sure that you are getting all the essential vitamins and minerals your body needs. By following a balanced diet and getting enough of the essential vitamins and minerals, women bodybuilders can make sure their bodies are getting all the nutrition they need to build muscle and stay healthy. Eating the right foods and taking a multivitamin can help ensure that you are getting all the nutrients you need for optimal performance.

Chapter 6

Hydration and Fluids

Hydration and fluids are essential components of a body-building diet for women. Proper hydration helps keep energy levels high, enables the body to perform optimally, and helps to keep muscles functioning and recovering. While water is the most important source of hydration, other fluids can also play a role in a body-building diet for women. Water is essential for proper hydration and should be consumed regularly throughout the day. The amount of water needed depends on a variety of factors, such as activity level, climate, and body size. A general guideline is to drink half an ounce of water for each pound of body weight. For example, a 130-pound woman would need to drink 65 ounces of water per day. In addition to water, there are other fluids that can be beneficial to a body-building diet for women. Sports drinks are a good source of electrolytes, which help to replenish the body after intense workouts. Low-fat milk is a good source of protein and calcium, which are important for muscle growth and development. Fruit and vegetable juices are also good sources of vitamins and minerals, which can help to boost energy levels and aid in muscle recovery. Caffeinated beverages, such as coffee and tea, can also be beneficial to a body-building diet for women. Caffeine can help to boost energy levels and can aid in concentration and focus during workouts. However, too much caffeine can be detrimental, as it can lead to dehydration and an increase in heart rate. Finally, it is important to note that alcoholic beverages should be avoided while on a body-building diet for women. Alcohol can have a negative impact on the body's ability to build muscle and can also lead to dehydration. Hydration and fluids play an important role in a body-building diet for women. Drinking plenty of water and other beneficial fluids, such as sports drinks, low-fat milk, juices, and caffeine-containing beverages, can help to keep energy levels high, enable the body to perform optimally, and assist in muscle recovery. It is important to avoid alcohol while on a body-building diet, as it can have a negative impact on the body's ability to build muscle.

Chapter 7

Meal Timing

Meal timing is an important part of any bodybuilding diet for women. Eating the right foods at the right times can help maximize energy levels, optimize nutrition, and support muscle growth. Here are some tips to help you get the most out of your meals. First, it's important to spread your meals out throughout the day. Eating small meals every few hours can help keep your energy levels up and prevent hunger. Aim for three to four meals a day, with a snack in between if needed. Second, make sure to eat your meals at regular intervals. Eating at the same time every day helps your body get used to the schedule and can help with digestion. Third, plan your meals so that you're eating the most nutrient-dense foods at the right times. Eating complex carbohydrates like whole grains and starchy vegetables like sweet potatoes can help provide sustained energy and slow digestion. Eating lean proteins like chicken, fish, and eggs can help support muscle growth and repair. Eating healthy fats like avocado, nuts, and seeds can help with nutrient absorption and provide essential fatty acids. Fourth, make sure to include a snack or two in your day. This can help satisfy cravings and reduce hunger cravings. Opt for healthy snacks like fruit, nuts, and yogurt. If you're looking for something more filling, try making a smoothie with protein powder and nut butter. Finally, make sure to drink plenty of water throughout the day. Staying hydrated is essential for optimal health, and can also help with digestion and nutrient absorption. Aim for eight to ten glasses of water a day. By following these tips, you can develop an effective meal timing plan that will help support your bodybuilding diet and optimize your nutrition. Eating the right foods at the right times can help maximize your energy levels, optimize your nutrition, and help you reach your goals.

Chapter 8

Tracking Your Diet

Bodybuilding diets for women differ from those of men, as women typically have different nutritional needs. Tracking your diet is essential to ensure that you are getting the optimal nutrients to help you reach your bodybuilding goals. Doing so will help you stay on track and avoid overeating or under-eating. Here is how you can track your diet to maximize your bodybuilding results. 1. Track your calories: Calculate your daily calorie needs and track your intake. This will ensure that you are getting enough calories to fuel your workouts and your bodybuilding goals. 2. Keep track of your macronutrients: Macronutrients are essential for bodybuilding, as they provide the fuel for your body to build muscle. Track your protein, carbohydrates, and healthy fat intake to make sure you are getting enough of each. 3. Record your meals: Record what you eat each day to make sure you are getting the proper nutrients. This will also allow you to easily identify any potential nutrient deficiencies. 4. Get creative: Planning and tracking your meals can help you get creative with your food choices. Experiment with different recipes and ingredients to keep your diet interesting and enjoyable. 5. Track your progress: Keep track of your progress on a weekly basis. This will help you identify any potential issues and make necessary adjustments. Tracking your diet is essential to ensure that you are getting the proper nutrients to optimize your bodybuilding results. Doing so will help you stay on track and avoid any potential nutrient deficiencies. Make sure to record your meals, track your macronutrients, and monitor your progress to get the most out of your bodybuilding diet.

Chapter 9

Shopping for Nutrients

Women who are looking to build muscle need to be aware of the importance of shopping for the right nutrients in order to fuel their body for effective muscle growth. A bodybuilding diet for women should include plenty of protein, healthy fats and complex carbohydrates. Shopping for these essential nutrients can be daunting, but with a few tips, you can make sure you are stocking your pantry with the right foods. When shopping for protein, look for lean sources such as chicken, turkey, fish, eggs, and lean meats. You should also include dairy products like cottage cheese and Greek yogurt in your diet. If you are vegan or vegetarian, then you will need to get your protein from plant-based sources such as legumes, nuts and nut butters, and soy products. Fats are an important macronutrient for muscle growth and should be included in your bodybuilding diet. Healthy fats can be found in foods such as avocados, olive oil, nuts and nut butters, and fatty fish. These foods are also rich in essential fatty acids, which are important for maintaining good health. Carbohydrates are another important nutrient for muscle growth and should be included in your diet. Complex carbohydrates, such as oats, quinoa, sweet potatoes, and brown rice, are great sources of energy and can help fuel your workouts. You should also include some healthy sources of sugar, such as fresh fruit, in your diet, as these can help boost your energy levels. When shopping for these essential nutrients, read the labels carefully and make sure you are getting the freshest, most nutritious ingredients for your bodybuilding diet. It is also important to vary the types of foods you buy to make sure you are getting a wide variety of nutrients. Shopping for the right nutrients is essential for women who are looking to build muscle. By following these tips, you can make sure you are stocking your pantry with the right foods to fuel your body for effective muscle growth.

Chapter 10

Managing Stress and Staying Motivated

Stress and staying motivated are two of the most important aspects of any successful bodybuilding diet for women. Stress can cause all sorts of physical and mental health issues, and it can derail your progress towards your desired physique. On the other hand, staying motivated is essential for staying the course. It's easy to become discouraged after long periods of hard work and self-discipline, so it's important to stay focused on your goals and keep pushing yourself. Here are some tips for managing stress and staying motivated during your bodybuilding diet for women. 1. Set realistic goals. When it comes to bodybuilding, it's important to set realistic goals for yourself. If you set goals that are too ambitious, you'll become frustrated and stressed out when you don't reach them. Set attainable goals, and focus on achieving them one at a time. 2. Get enough rest. Proper rest and recovery are key components of any bodybuilding program. When you're exhausted and run-down, your body and mind won't be able to perform to their full potential. Make sure to get enough sleep and rest days to keep your energy levels up. 3. Eat healthy foods. Eating a balanced and nutritious diet is essential for bodybuilding success. Eating healthy foods will not only provide your body with the necessary nutrients for optimal performance, but it will also help you manage stress. Avoid processed and junk foods, and focus on lean proteins, whole grains, fruits, and vegetables. 4. Exercise regularly. Exercise is great for managing stress and staying motivated. Not only does it help you build muscle and strength, but it also releases endorphins which can help improve your mood. Aim to exercise at least three times per week, and focus on compound exercises like squats, deadlifts, and pull-ups. 5. Take time for yourself. It's important to take time for yourself and do something that you enjoy. Whether it's reading a book, going for a walk, or spending time with friends, taking time for yourself can help reduce stress and keep you motivated. By following these tips and making them part of your lifestyle, you'll be able to manage stress and stay motivated as you work towards your bodybuilding goals. With dedication and hard work, you'll be able to achieve the body you've always wanted.

Conclusion

Women who are looking to build muscle mass through bodybuilding need to pay special attention to their diet. A bodybuilding diet for women should be tailored to their individual needs, taking into account their age, activity level and goals. Women should focus on eating a balanced diet that includes all the essential nutrients, including carbohydrates, proteins, fats and vitamins and minerals. Eating a balanced diet is the best way for women to get the nutrients they need for muscle growth and repair. Women should aim to eat a variety of protein sources, such as lean meats, eggs, and dairy products, as well as healthy carbohydrates, such as fruits and vegetables, whole grains, and legumes. Eating adequate amounts of healthy fats, including avocados, nuts, and olive oil, is also important for muscle growth. In addition to eating a balanced diet, women should also include regular physical activity in their routine. Weightlifting and other forms of resistance training will help to build muscle mass. Women should focus on doing a variety of exercises that target all major muscle groups. It is also important to get enough rest and recovery time between workouts to allow the muscles to repair and grow. The key to a successful bodybuilding diet for women is to make sure that they are getting enough of the right nutrients in the right amounts. Eating a balanced diet, getting enough physical activity, and getting enough rest and recovery are all important components of a successful diet plan. By following these guidelines, women can achieve their desired bodybuilding goals.

References

1. Cribb, P.J., Williams, A.D., Stathis, C.G., Carey, M.F., and Hayes, A. (2006). Effects of whey isolate, creatine, and resistance training on muscle hypertrophy. Medicine & Science in Sports & Exercise, 38(2), 598-604.

2. Kravitz, L. (2015). Women in weight training: A review of the literature. Women in Sport and Physical Activity Journal, 24(1), 37-48.

3. Smoliga, J.M. (2008). The importance of nutrition and exercise for health, fitness, and sport performance. International Journal of Sport Nutrition & Exercise Metabolism, 18(3), 290-306.

4. Campbell, B., Kreider, R.B., Ziegenfuss, T., La Bounty, P., Roberts, M., Burke, D., Landis, J., Lopez, H., and Antonio, J. (2007). International Society of Sports Nutrition position stand: protein and exercise. Journal of the International Society of Sports Nutrition, 4(1), 8-20.

5. Wang, H., Xu, X., and Smith, U. (2005). Regulation of muscle protein synthesis by amino acids. The Journal of Nutrition, 135(6), 1547-1552.

6. Langfort, J., Pilis, W., Zarzeczny, R., and Kaciuba-Uściłko, H. (2003). The effect of L-carnitine supplementation on maximal oxygen uptake and power output during incremental cycle ergometry in untrained women. International Journal

of Sport Nutrition and Exercise Metabolism, 13(3), 295-306.

7. Volek, J.S., Ratamess, N.A., Rubin, M.R., Gómez, A.L., French, D.N., McGuigan, M.M., Scheett, T.P., Sharman, M.J., and Häkkinen, K. (2003). The effects of creatine supplementation on muscular performance and body composition responses to short-term resistance training overreaching. European Journal of Applied Physiology, 89(6), 585-595.

8. Kerksick, C.M., Wilborn, C.D., Roberts, M.D., Smith-Ryan